HOW TO STAY SLIM ONE BITE AT A TIME

HOW TO STAY SLIM ONE BITE AT A TIME

SONIA HANSBERRY

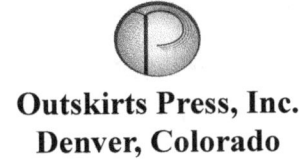

Outskirts Press, Inc.
Denver, Colorado

Table of Contents

Dedication

This book is dedicated to my wonderful mom and dad, who raised me to be a woman of integrity. Their love, joy, and kindness have always been there for me. I love you with all my heart.

Mom, thank you for your words of wisdom. I look at my mom and say, "Wow." She is a beautiful and loving mother. She always told me "Take care of your body and your body will be around for a long time". Mom, I will always admire your style and poise. In my eyes, you are a prime example of a wonderful mom. Her motto is, "Do everything in moderation."

Foreword

Do you really want to know how I stay slim, one bite at a time? Well, I can honestly say: it is truly one bite at a time!

For one, I know when it is time to stop eating when my stomach says I am full! I also don't eat all of my food. This is not by choice; rather, I have always been that way, and did not realize that by eating this way, I kept my weight down until I read a magazine article about how most Europeans eat small portions. These small portions are filled with some of the richest nutrients and finest ingredients in the world. Since the food is rich in nutrients, it does the body good, Therefore, the food is prepared well and nourishes your body so you won't overeat.

I am here to tell you that you can eat small portions , too, regardless of what race, creed or color you are. Here are some tips that I have learned over the years.

You can balance your food intake, whether it is rich in nutrients or not like fast food. The number one thing is to eat small portions.

Now, this may not be easy for some, or even most. For instance, some people were raised in large families; therefore, they ate as much as they could, so no one else would get it. Other people just like to eat. Still others were raised in the South, and this was how they learned to cook from Mom. Well, let me tell you, home-cooked, and fast food is not the same as it was ten to fifteen years ago. It definitely has more stuff in it than it did twenty years ago. Trust me you can change with just a little willpower day in and day out, just eat small portions. Once again, balance your eating.

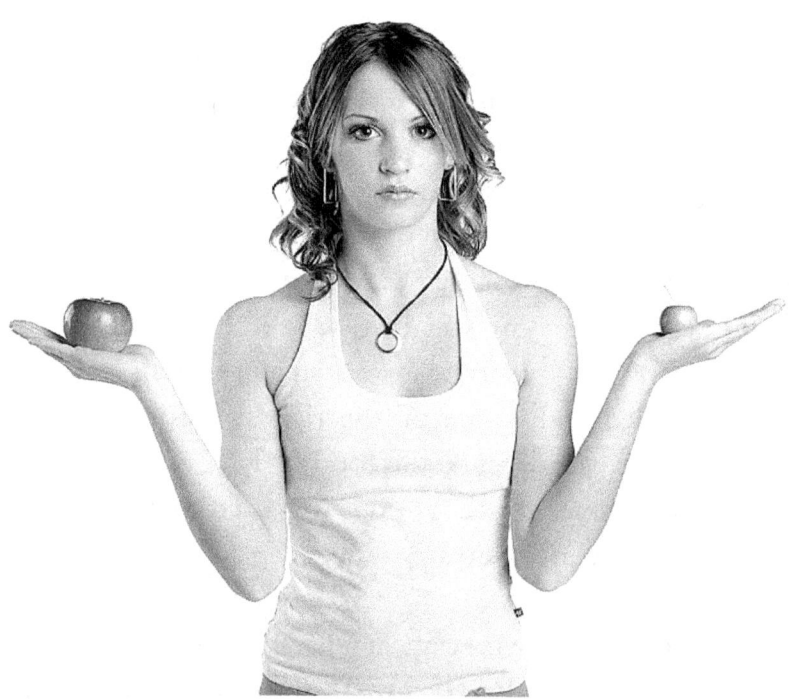

Think to yourself as you are ordering fast food, "Do I need to supersize this No. 12 meal? Do I need twelve nuggets versus six nuggets or even three nuggets? Do I need those fries?" This is where it hurts—the fries, one of the most damaging items on any fast-food menu. The fries alone can knock anybody's eating habits out the ballpark. But at the same time, just because there are fifty fries in the box doesn't mean you have to eat all of them. It is called common sense. I know what you are thinking: Who eats three nuggets? Well, I do. Once again, I have acquired this eating habit over the years, so it is normal for me! If not, try to scale back until your body desires to eat small portions again. At the same, time you have to balance your sweet tooth. The sugar is the thing that sits in your body over-night and creates fat.

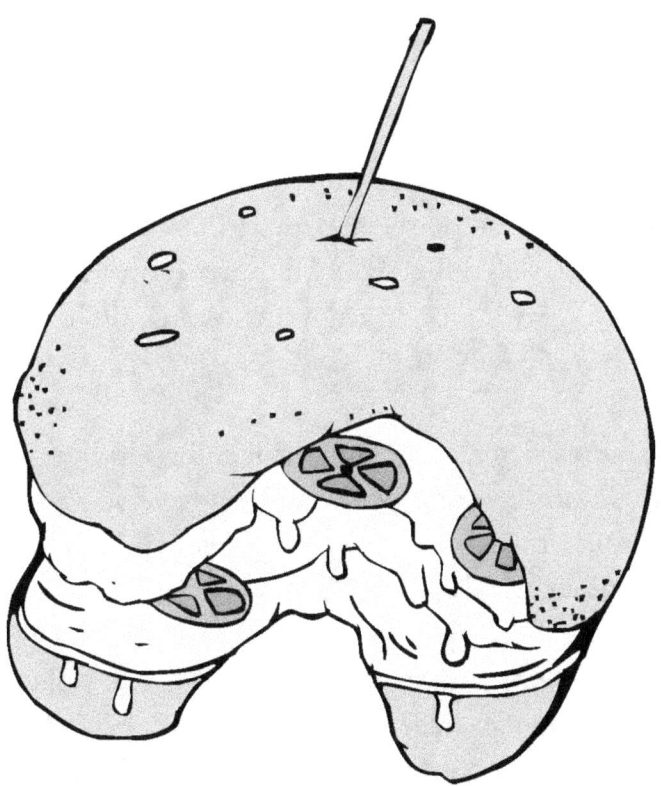

I know what you are thinking: What if I am still hungry? Well, grab some water and/or a low-fat snack. If you choose a high-calorie snack, once again, eat in moderation; that is the key. If you get hungry at night before bed, I suggest drinking water and/or a hot cup of honey and cinnamon. This will reduce the hunger pains and it is also good for your body. As we all know, most people after age thirty-five, and even more so after forty, should not be eating later than 7 p.m. on a normal workday evening. There are those times where you are at a restaurant, and you may eat a late Friday night or Saturday night dinner, but once again, eat in moderation; instead of that Pepsi, drink water instead.

I guarantee that if you use this tactic with your entire food intake, take up a simple form of exercise, such as walking and/ or using a treadmill, and drink plenty of water, you will notice a significant change in your midsection within weeks. Some people differ; you may lose it on your buttocks and/or your thighs. Of course, this is based on how your body was created in the first place. Put it this way: by eating like this, you will see a drop in your clothing size, leaving you with a body ready for toning. Of course, all this depends on your metabolism.

If you get hungry later, grab some fruit and go to bed. There is no reason for you to be eating before you go to bed. You can try this tactic for about a month and lose weight instantly. Exercising is also good. Remember, it's always better to exercise with a partner.

In the morning, eat something light, such as one boiled egg, one piece of toast, orange juice and/or coffee. For lunch, eat a half of a sandwich, a few chips, and a soda. For dinner, eat one piece of chicken and a few vegetables. You can actually count them: ten peas, ten string beans, four pieces of broccoli, etc.

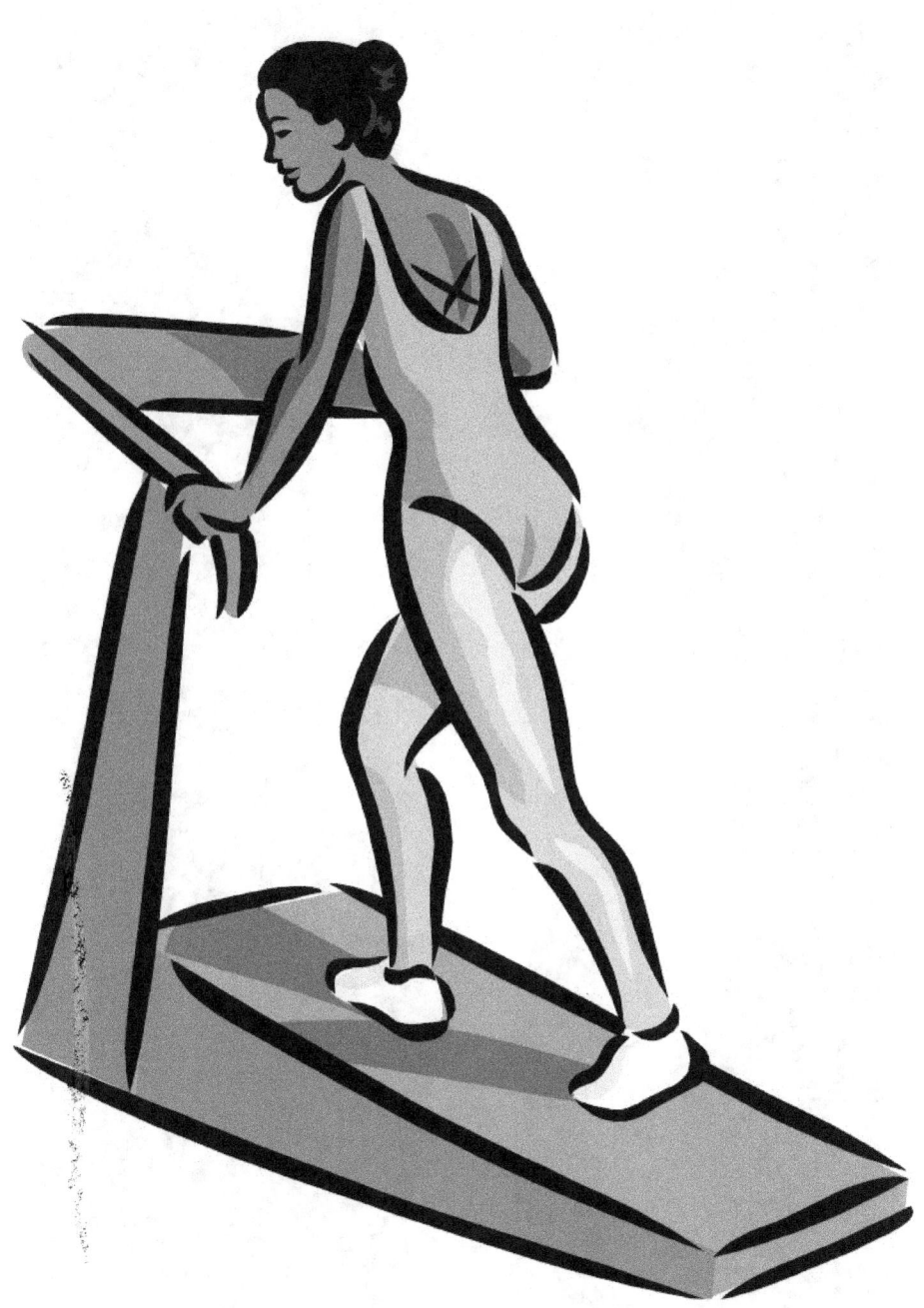

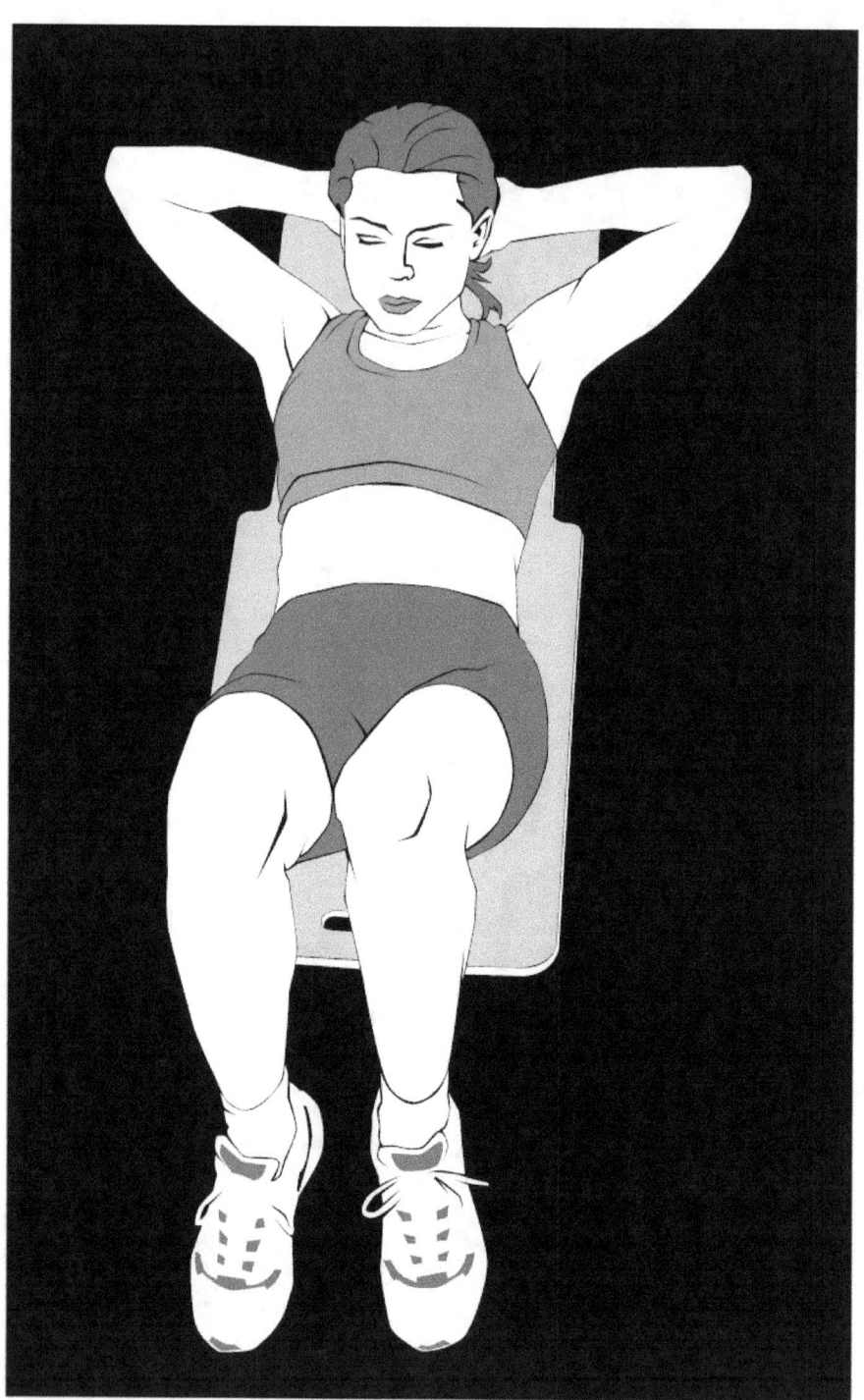

JUST EAT SMALL PORTIONS!

Females go through changes where they may binge during their menstrual cycle. That's okay; go ahead and binge, but when you binge on your favorite foods, eat less of them. Try to stay away from the sugar.

In my early twenties, the rumor was to go out to lunch with Sonia. Well, I found out why! People could order a large meal, eat the majority of the food, and split the cost with me. Their advantage was to eat more food and save money; my advantage was to get a small meal without wasting it. My family and friends knew that even if they shared with me, they would end up getting more. This was a win-win situation for everyone.

I would basically share anything with anybody. Once again, this was not by choice, not by accident, and not because I wanted to lose weight and/or stay slim. This was just something in my genes. It made me think of a combination of my giving nature and staying slim at the same time. Believe me, there were times when people did not want to share, but I would continue my habit of ordering

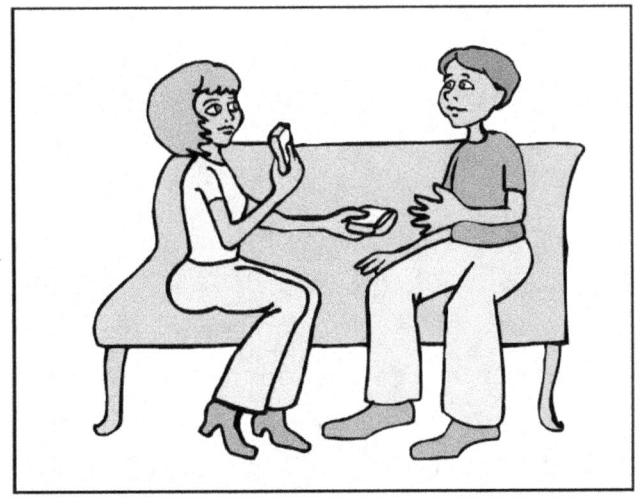

appetizers and/or items off the kids' meal menu (if I could get away with it).

Several times I would have to take a doggy bag even with small portions. Then one day I got smart: I would ask the server to give me way less on my plate than usually came with the dish.

Now when it came to desserts—and we know how expensive that is—I would also share. Sometimes, I did not want to spend the average six to eight bucks for dessert at a restaurant, knowing it was fattening at the same time. Therefore, I would wait until I got home or back to the office and get me a bag of M&Ms and peanut chews. I would eat maybe two, and save the rest for the remainder of the week. This satisfied my sweet tooth.

I would also ask the waitress for a small portion. This allows me to eat just enough; too much food on my plate puts me off eating. I am considered a pack rat when it comes to sweets. I would have some potato chips with my sandwich, eat half of a small bag, and save the rest for the next day. If I am at work and I have a sweet tooth, I stake out the candy dishes. I savor that one bite-size Snickers one little bite at a time, and enjoy it like it was a king-size candy bar. This would satisfy my craving, while at the same time cut back on the calories.

I did not realize I had such strange habits until my daughter told me, "Ma, you eat like a little mouse."

She said she had never seen anybody eat the way I do. I guess that people who did not know me, who would see me at different functions where I would not eat all of my food thought I was doing this on purpose. My eating habits were never a conscious choice. I haven't told you about the slow eating; yep, it takes me at least an hour to eat my food. Once again, I did this without realizing what I was doing.

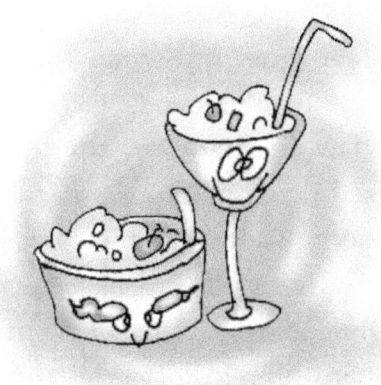

This also contributed to me staying slim by giving my food time to digest. I will never forget a time when I was about thirty years old when someone approached me and said, "Stop faking and eat all of your food!" I said, "Excuse me!" She said, "Now I know how you stay so slim" and told me my secret was exposed. This situation was very strange to me, but very amusing!

The amusing part was that someone would be paying that much attention to me at a luncheon where the concentration should be on enjoying the company of family and friends. Once I had gotten over the strangeness, I said, "Excuse me, I have no idea what you are talking about. And anyway, why are you watching me so closely anyway?"

We laughed it off later, and I told her that these had been my eating habits my whole life. She asked me to help her with her eating habits. After I discussed my techniques with her, she took my advice, lost weight, and started exercising. She made it part of her daily regimen. Even now, she still teases me about that moment when she told me off!

People always ask me what my secret to staying slim is. Once I reveal to them some of the things I see that are hurting them, for the most part they listen and my advice works for them. Most of them are shocked that I am aware of their eating habits. With women who are sincere, I spend a little more time telling them how they can lose weight. By this time, I have become aware of my co-workers' eating habits and have to tell them the truth about why they are having a hard time losing weight and/or getting ready to go up into another size.

Once I reveal to them some of the things I see that are hurting them, they, for the most part, listen, and my advice works for them. Most of them are shocked that I am aware of their eating habits. I don't watch them; it is just that I am aware of my surroundings most of the time. I would also be shocked if someone told me how often I eat certain unhealthy things. Once again, if someone offers you a doughnut or a piece of cake, eat only half and/or take several bites just to satisfy your craving.

The moral of this story is that some people like to eat, and other people overindulge for various reasons—upbringing, depression, etc.

We have to stop the excuses. Push away from the table! Don't go back for seconds.

I have also had men ask me what my secret is. This one guy would actually come to my desk just to see what I was eating, so he could try and do the same thing to lose weight. I was able to give him some helpful hints.

When my daughter cooks spaghetti and meatballs, she tells me, "You get one meatball, about five strands of spaghetti, and for dessert you get one cookie and/or one scoop of ice cream." She finds this very amusing. Yes, this is true. She has also adopted my eating habits!

Don't get me wrong; you will gain weight as you age and your metabolism decreases. But remember: moderation is the key. Personally, I would rather have a moderate exercise regimen, eat right, and gain weight naturally rather than gaining weight by overeating. Trust me, as you begin to adapt to this habit your stomach will get used to small portions, and then your brain will automatically tell you when your stomach is full. You will have gained control over food, instead of food gaining control over you.

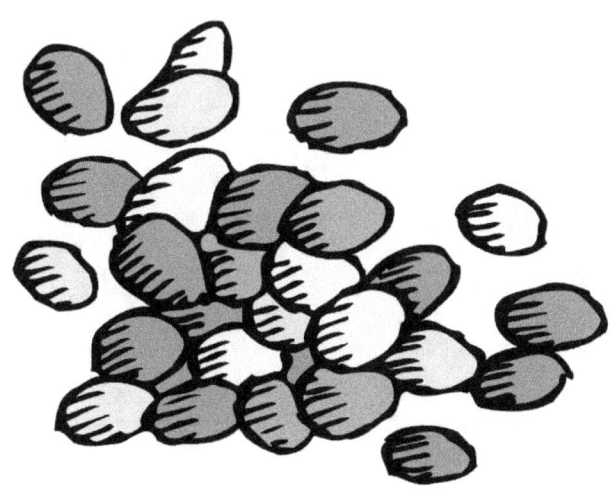

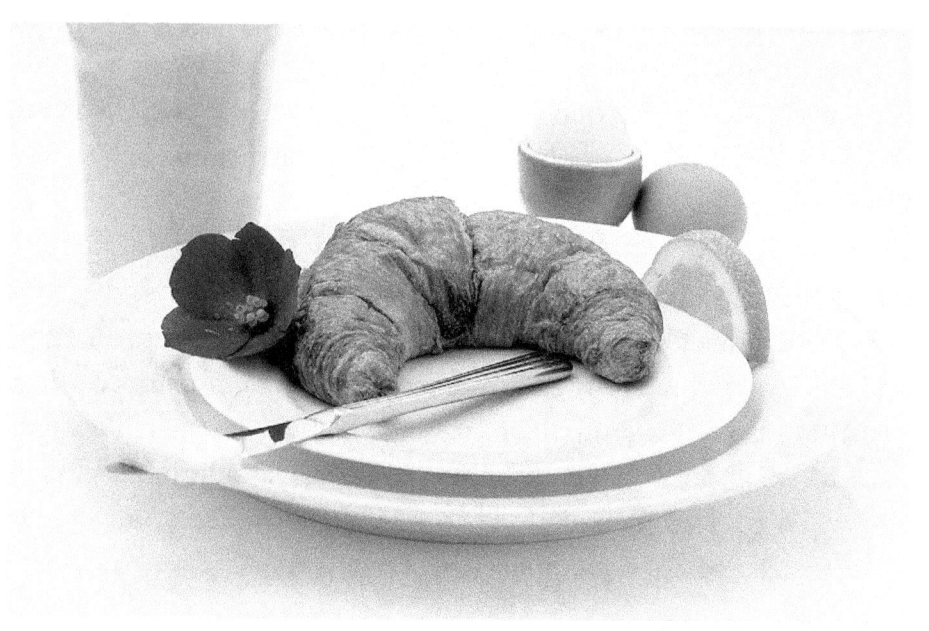

Tips on How to Get Fit and Stay Healthy

1. What Is Your Body Saying?

First of all, I have to admit there are all shapes and sizes. There are plenty of diets and exercise programs, and I find that people who go in for these kinds of programs tend to be gluttons for punishment. With a little common sense and exercise, anyone can maintain their desired weight and stay healthy—and that includes staying away from the doctor's office. I honestly believe if a person becomes in tune with their body, they can maintain a healthy, slim, trim body in accordance with their general makeup—basically, the way you were created. Everybody is different; therefore, you have to be realistic and know your own body. This includes your metabolism, your structure, and your genes. It is important to get to know your body. Just remember your body is your temple, and what you put into it will become a part of you. Therefore, instead of struggling to be or look like someone else, get to know your own body; this will eliminate a lot of frustration.

2. How to Stay Slim

Read the Entire Book.

3. Lose Ten Pounds in Ten Days

I know you have seen these commercials. Crashing does not help you. You have to wean yourself from your old habits. You have to cut back, eat healthier, and be determined. If you keep to this process you will see a difference in about three to four weeks.

4. Dreaming of Eating Instead of Cows

Food can become very addictive, especially during stressful times. If you direct your energy toward eating good food, your body will give you sufficient energy. We all have to eat, but the key is obtaining the nutrition and calories you need to survive and also to thrive.

5. Depression Eating

I believe half of all Americans are affected by this issue. We always blame it on our past, our bone structure, how our parents fed us, hunger while we were growing up, and the famous one—just plain comfort food. These are all lies you are telling yourself. When you find yourself pigging out for no reason at all, stop, listen, and think. Ask yourself, "What am I doing?" Once you identify this bad habit you can take the first step toward a healthier, more productive way of eating. Also, you may want to call someone to help you through that moment. All these reasons will definitely hold you back from a successful plan of maintaining healthy habits. This concept reminds me of a drafty window. Until you find the draft, the wind will forever whirl you away into food land.

6. Be Yourself

Let's face it, I am not a nutritionist, but I have the nutritional common sense to know a piece of toast is far better than a doughnut in the morning. But don't just stick to some boring breakfast, lunch, and dinner plan. Read and educate yourself on your favorite foods; learn to make them with less dressing, less butter, less of everything. The more you know about food and what it has to offer your body, the better able you will be to create a plan just for you. Yes, you! You were designed differently from everyone else; therefore, you need to custom-design an eating plan that will work for you. This may take a couple of tries. The key is to be consistent. Consistency brings results. Just don't give up.

7. 'Come on, I Know this Nice Restaurant'

You have heard this before. Either it is your pocketbook that does not want to go or it is your diet plan you worked so hard to maintain! Changing your eating habits is just as important as losing the weight. This is one of those moments where you have to tell your friends what you are trying to accomplish. A true friend will support you. Your willpower will allow you to do what's best for you. Eventually, you will look good; once this happens, your friends will respect you—not to mention also wanting to follow your regimen.

8. The I See, See, Eat, Eat Balancing Act!

Oh boy! This is a tough one. At one time during our earlier years, we were able to eat and eat. Then we were able to eat and do a little exercise. Well, that combination becomes more like eat right and exercise daily after your mid-thirties. During this time of your life, it is important to burn as many calories as possible.

HOW TO STAY SLIM ONE BITE AT A TIME

Losing weight and weight control have a lot to do with the number of calories consumed versus calories burned in your body. If you eat more calories than your body has burned, your body will retain the fuel as fat to be burned when it is needed. On the other hand, if you take in the same number of calories that you burn, your body will draw on stored energy—fat—and burn it up to keep it going. The amount of calories needed by your body depends on gender, age, build, metabolism and—most importantly—your activity level.

When you are active, you burn more calories than when you are sedentary. All other factors being equal, it takes a 130-pound person approximately thirty calories to sit and watch TV for a half hour. Doing desk work for the same duration burns twice that number. Play a rousing game of ping-pong and the ante is upped to about a hundred calories. Walk two miles in that half hour and the calorie consumption is raised to something closer to 160. Thirty minutes of climbing stairs burns a fabulous 440 calories.

It's is no secret that when you are active you burn more calories than just sitting around. Sitting down and watching TV takes about thirty calories, but reading the newspaper will burn twice that much. If you play a game of pool you are talking about approximately a hundred calories. Walking and climbing stairs burns approximately five hundred calories.

The above example not only burns the calories, but also builds a greater rate of calories in general. Basically, they are considered bonus calories as a result of the exercise. It reminds me of reward points on a credit card: every time you charge an item, you get reward points.

When you make exercise or some other activity a part of your life, it will diminish your appetite. The best part is that this discourages overeating.

I find that after a brisk walk I feel a noticeable lift in my mood. Because many people overeat to offset feelings of boredom, sadness, or loneliness, that mood change will offer a positive effect on weight loss as well. Your sense of well-being will depend less on food, and you will learn to eat only due to actual hunger. Therefore, watch what you eat, and count calories if this helps. Keep in mind that it is great to exercise and eat right, but just remember that success really happens when you pay as much attention to exercise as you do diet.

9. I Was Raised on Collard Greens, Cakes, Pies, and Mashed Potatoes. What Do I Do Now?

How many times have you heard this excuse? People are quick to use this excuse for explaining problems with losing weight and why they gain weight. Their mentality is, "Since my mom and dad fed me like that thirty years ago, I will continue to eat like that, including feeding my kids the same way." Most of childhood has close emotional associations with family history.

Now, for me, it was my sweet tooth that was my parents' downfall. Even to this day my mom still desires something sweet after dinner. Therefore, my sister and I developed the same habit. This was fine for me about ten years ago. Now it is three Oreos and 2-percent-fat milk, whereas ten years ago it was ten Oreo cookies and a full glass of whole milk. The point is not to toss the old out, but rather to make realistic, conscious choices. If childhood habits serve your adult priorities, enjoy them to the full. If they get in your way, acknowledge the need to look for new options.

10. You Will Know When it is Time to Eat

People associate eating with your stomach growling. When you feel your stomach growling, wait at least ten minutes before responding. If this technique does not work, still wait and see. If hunger still persists after you drink a large glass of water, then eat some fruit and/or a high-energy snack. Fruits, low-fat yogurt, almonds, or a couple of crackers are good high-energy snacks. Drink one more glass of water. If you are used to eating high-fat processed snacks, the whole natural-food regimen may not be appealing. For the most part, people have found that high-calorie snacks do not satisfy their energy needs without leading to more cravings.

11. Be Realistic with Your Decisions

Any time you are faced with the challenge of losing several pounds, it can seem much more realistic over a period of time. Dieting and exercising is new to you and you need to pace yourself. Set small goals. I would cut everything in half. With exercise, start out gradually, and then build up to your full potential. Repeat this process; you will eventually get used to it. The weight loss will add up before you know it. Eventually you will realize how much power you actually have to make the life that you want.

12. Forgive Yourself

Don't beat yourself up. There will be days when your eating and exercise plan will feel unbearable. Whenever change occurs, we have to adapt to it. It all starts with your attitude: if you get down on yourself, you will lose confidence, and your confidence level will short-circuit your hopes and goals.

The key to unlock your power is to realize you are only human. You are going to make mistakes, and the majority of those mistakes will be rebellious moments of eating what you want and not exercising. But remember you can only change on the basis of your undesirable experiences. Therefore, forgive yourself if you get off the track. Live and learn. Basically, draw a bridge and get over it.

13. Watch Food-Centered Socializing

This will definitely either make or break your desired weight and exercise regimen! Food, family and friends, sharing meals, cooking together—these are part of mealtime rituals.

This really creates a problem when you have a busy social calendar. Most of the time, the gatherings are comprised of fattening foods and alcohol. Therefore, the key is to measure how much socializing you do. Remember, everything in moderation; you always have a choice—pick the best one for you.

14. Quality of Food, Not Quantity

Are you happy with your weight? Well, you have to get a grip on what you eat; it really does matter.

The rise in obesity has been dramatic. I believe this stems from fast food, high-sugar foods, and less nutritional packaged foods. Even though people see the negative effects, they still tend to ignore the facts.

Have you noticed that people eat low- or no-fat foods in far larger portions than necessary because they believe that lack of fat means quantity no longer matters? This is also a myth with diet desserts and snacks. They do contain less fat or sugar, but the calories still linger. Don't be fooled by the box; you cannot eat the entire box and not gain weight—you will gain weight! Therefore, eat a well-balanced meal comprising a good combination of meat, fruit, and vegetables. Once again, you only need an adequate amount. Once you educate yourself on the proper calorie intake for your size, gender, and activity level, coupled with a well-rounded diet, you can take yourself off the "overweight" list. Common sense is, don't eat more than you need to eat.

It is interesting to know that, in the present age of diet soda, no-fat goodies, and numerous weight-loss programs and publications, the rise in obesity is dramatic. This is definitely a problem that stems from people who eat high-fat and high-sugar foods, fast food, and an overload of nutrition-less packaged food.

Despite all of the information on the negative effects of such a diet, people tend to ignore the facts.

15. Eat Small Portions, but Don't Forget Nutrition

How many times have you seen the human nutritional needs published by the US government? In school, at your job, the cafeteria, weight loss centers—it comes up everywhere. Well, this information will not help you unless you understand it as well as use it in your own exercise plan and daily eating habits.

Lack of knowledge is the No. 1 reason we fail to maintain a healthy-eating lifestyle. You have to read about nutrition to gain a better understanding of how to turn your hopes for a healthy and fit body into reality.

Read up on the nutrition, get sound current advice, and focus on a concentrated study until you know the facts so well that they become second nature to you.

Make a commitment to that eating style for a least a month. Just imagine: if you replace a nutrition-poor diet with one that follows informed guidelines, I guarantee you will experience positive returns in your vitality, weight control, and, most of all, self-esteem.

Remember, your body has to have a balance of nutrients to function efficiently and healthily. These are some of the reasons it might not be working well:

Eating food with poor nutrients.

The improper nutrients may contribute to a weight problem and other health-related difficulties.

Your body continues to demand food.

You feel a desire to eat, despite the fact that your have consumed as many or more calories than you require.

You continue to eat, not satisfying the real need your hunger represents.

Therefore, you eat more, and on and on. You can readily imagine where this cycle leads.

Finally, you reach the point of physical and psychological deprivation, leading to overeating.

16. Learn How to Stop Eating—Just Say No!

Why can't we just say no to food? We know our bellies are full and we continue to eat. Well, this has to stop. You have to identify the common-sense rules that apply to your worst eating habits and take steps to change them.

I can hear the excuse now! "My mom told me not to waste food," or, "We would not have healthy, strong bones if we did not eat all of our food." Is it not amazing how the habits learned early in our lives settles into a mindset for a lifetime? Of course, our caloric needs were high and our activity was constant. Unfortunately, we continued that style of eating not because our needs have remained the same, but because the habits have a pleasant association with our families.

Another problem is that we eat too fast; we are always in a hurry to get to a meeting, to pick the kids up, to meet the deadline. We only have half an hour for school or work lunch. This creates havoc in our system, which does not have enough time to register that we have eaten what we need—therefore, the brains says "eat more." As I mentioned above, I also ate slowly. I did not know these things mattered, but they sure helped me as I got older.

Whatever your reason for overeating is, stop. You have to come up with a better strategy. Therefore, a good suggestion is to put less on your plate, and don't even think about seconds. If you are being served, tell the person to limit the portions.

Don't eat so fast. Chew your food thoroughly. About a half hour before mealtime, drink a large glass of water so that you don't attack your meal. This way your stomach will not feel as empty.

I imagine you are saying, "Yeah right, a glass of water will not help me." Well, I did not say it was going to be easy. Remember, these simple strategies do require a lot of self-knowledge and a clear view of what you eat in the long run. The problem is not learning how to stop eating, but, like everything else in life, it is a learning process.

17. Oh No! Special Occasions: Birthday Parties, Christmas Parties, Office Parties, and More

The holiday season is the most damaging time of year, but it is also the best time of year to exercise your willpower.

If you master these events, you have won half the battle. The secret is to be one step ahead of the occasion. This means that, in weeks, months, or days, eat right, and exercise diligently. Once you are at the function, you will enjoy the occasion and avoid overeating.

Don't fall for thinking that this is a grueling regimen you have to do every day; look at it as a regimen that will add joy to your life, reduce stress, and result in better doctor reports. Life is too short to let happy occasions pass us by or undermine our goals.

18. Today, Tomorrow, Yesterday

Tell yourself "just for today" day by day for a week or two, and you'll have made a good start toward reaching your goals. Your daily success will gain momentum and help motivate you for each day going forward. You'll be on the way to gaining an excellent tool for managing procrastination in other areas of your life.

19. Come Out of the Closet and Leave the Doughnuts Behind

You have to be honest about secret eating. Once you recognize this behavior, you need to let someone know. Once you admit to the habit, it will no longer be a secret. So don't give into the eating impulse; take charge of the closet, keep it closed, and continue to discover the changes you are in the process of making.

20. Whole Versus Processed Foods

I believe the majority of the population is guilty of eating pre-packaged foods, whether for an easy dinner, easy lunch, or easy breakfast—or all three. Pop it in the microwave oven for three to five minutes and you are on your way to processed heaven, calories, and excessive salt intake.

You have to realize, when you set out on an eating plan, that you will become bored with it. Therefore, establish a set of better habits that will make sure your "weight loss" days come to an end. You want to be able to sustain your desired weight just by eating more natural foods.

21. Take Your Hand off the Trigger

We all have some type of associations with certain activities: movies—popcorn and soda; family board games—soda, chips, and candy; kids games—soda, popcorn, chicken; and the infamous watching television—dinner, ice cream, and cake or pie for dessert. These are moments you eat more than you want or need. These are considered "conditional eatings." Once you realize this, the key is to choose and eat better quality food. Don't fool yourself into thinking you can't stop this madness. You can change; the main thing is recognizing it and understanding what is taking place during these moments.

22. The Pantry Is Not Your Friend—Rethink Your Relationship

The pantry can sometimes be used as an excuse to keep our favorite treats on hand. The power of self-deception can be as strong as the power of positive thinking. You have to be your own critic when assessing your situation. Tell yourself, "I know it is painful," but face yourself and continue to strategize with authority and courage. You should no longer be scared to look in your pantry.

23. Boredom Eating—Avoid It

Boredom eating simply gratifies the need for something to do. You are eating because you are bored, procrastinating about something, too tired to fix a decent meal, or are balking at your new regimen.

All theses excuses lead to boredom eating. You have to pay attention to boredom all the time. Sometimes it is plain laziness, but there is hope. Therefore, you just need a little spark. Get off the sofa, put the ice cream away, and get busy doing an activity that means something to you. Eventually, food will no longer call your name or talk to you.

24. Talk to Yourself

I often talk to myself, especially when it comes to sweets. I am my own worst critic, while everyone is saying, "Oh go ahead, you know it is not going to hurt you." But my concern is the long run; I also have to be aware of the yellow brick sweet road. It is good to be your own worst critic as well as your own self-motivator. Believe me, life will offer you plenty of criticism; just make sure you are not the one doing it. Be yourself, and do what's right for you and your body.

25. Draw a Bridge and Get over It Fast

Okay, you have read the book and you say, "What"? You said you are going to get your weight under control and keep it under control. You have established some positive, realistic goals for change in your exercise and eating habits. Based on my experience, in three to five weeks, habits can be broken. All you have to do is apply yourself to several weeks of constant self-talk, self-motivation, and self-conscious consistency that will be helpful over your lifetime. You will notice a new you. You will view your new body and strength of purpose and then forget about it and enjoy life.

The 16 Most Common Questions, I Get Asked

1. How can I exercise, eat right, and lose weight at the same time?
2. What should I eat?
3. Do I have to cut out my favorite foods?
4. How do I get rid of baby fat?
5. How often should I work out?
6. What is good to eat for breakfast instead of fast food?
7. How do I get rid of my midsection?
8. How do I count calories?
9. Do my genes have anything to do with my weight?
10. What is the best exercise for my thighs?
11. Does a Diet Coke really work with my double cheeseburger?
12. How much should I eat?
13. How do I train my stomach to take in a little bit of food when I am used to gorging myself?
14. What is the best diet food?
15. When should I push away from the table?
16. When should I skip dessert?

HOW TO STAY SLIM ONE BITE AT A TIME

1. How can I exercise, eat right, and lose weight at the same time?

All you have to do is thirty minutes, at least three times a week. If thirty minutes is too much, do a quick fifteen minutes per day on your treadmill and/or some type of aerobic exercise. But make sure it's for at least fifteen minutes, three days a week. Actually, you do not have to exercise every day. *TIP:* If you are too busy and/or too lazy to exercise, then you need to make sure you eat the right foods in moderation.

2. What should I eat?

I basically eat what I want, anytime I want. The key is to eat the most nutritional foods the majority of the time. Most of the time I eat the normal breakfast, lunch, and dinner. *TIP*: If you decide to go beyond a nutritional snack such as fruit, nuts, raisins, etc., and purchase vending-machine snacks, then I suggest eating just part of the item and saving the rest for later.

3. Do I have to cut out my favorite foods?

No, you don't. But if your favorite food is Oreo cookies, fried chicken, meat loaf, pizza, or potatoes, just cut back on your servings. Eat more vegetables than the meat. *TIP: Whatever portion you normally eat, cut it in half; eat* two wings instead of ten; instead of five meatballs eat two meatballs. Don't try to eat the whole pizza; eat only two slices. When you order a pizza, order nutritional toppings, such as mushrooms, tomatoes, green peppers, etc. Treat your sweet tooth the same way. Instead of six cookies, eat two; instead of the pint of ice cream, have three huge spoonfuls; instead of the entire bag of chips, eat a handful.

4. How do I get rid of baby fat?

The baby fat may require a bit more scaling back as well as some type of sit-ups, crunches, etc. to tighten up your abdominal muscles. It takes a combination of healthy eating and exercise to lose your midsection. Here are five foolproof strategies to shed the baby fat.

TIP: Have you notice plates are huge? Well, personally I don't like to eat on huge plates. I prefer a smaller plate; it helps me to look at my food as a necessity to fulfill the hunger pains and not overindulge myself, especially if it is my favorite food. If you are at a restaurant and they fix large portions, once again, it does not mean you have to eat everything on your plate. If you go to a buffet, you definitely need to exercise self-control.

TIP: When I was pregnant, I ate a lot of vegetables. Since I was trying to lose the baby fat, I knew they had fewer calories than any other food item. Also, the high fiber made me feel full. This is definitely a sure way to reduce you calorie intake.

TIP: Make an exercise date. More than likely it will be you initiating this. I find once you start relying on others to hang out with you and exercise, their determination may be different from yours. Therefore, make a date with yourself. Today, all moms are busy, either working and/or taking care of children. If you have any time to yourself, take an exercise class, even if it is one day a week. For some moms, this is tough but if you start some type of exercise regimen now, that is less baby fat that has to come off when you go back to work. Once you go back to work, your normal schedule will go back to coming home, feeding and washing the baby, eating, and going to bed. Now you have another problem—the baby fat you are trying to get rid of, including the eating and zero exercise. The best way to beat this boring regimen is to put the baby in the stroller and go for a walk. I know that, "if there is a will there is a way!"

5. How often should I work out?

You should work out every day, if possible, while still watching your intake of food, especially sweets. After a certain age, it becomes imperative that you do a lot of exercising and a lot of cutting back on your favorite foods. It is better to do both; the exercise will energize your brain cells, and you think better and feel better when the heart rate is pumping. Trust me: with this regimen on a consistent basis (no cheating) you will definitely see results soon!

6. What is good to eat for breakfast instead of fast food?

I find, once again, it is okay to eat what you want for breakfast. I would not eat any doughnuts, cakes, or other pastries for breakfast, or anything with too much sugar. I would prefer some oatmeal, grits and toast, one boiled egg, two slices of toast, bananas, and/or any type of fruit or yogurt.

7. How do I get rid of my midsection?

This is a major problem for many people: the "pocket belly." It is the part of the body that makes or breaks our clothing. I don't believe all of us will ever have a super-flat stomach, but you can greatly improve your abdominal area and can end up with a sexy midsection that suits your body type just fine.

Midsection tips include:

- In your workout program, each week perform different abdominal exercises. This system is effective in keeping your abdominal muscles constantly challenged, which speeds up results.
- Eating habits are just as critical to leaning up your midsection. Replace sodium, sugar, and preservatives-laden foods with fresh, whole, unprocessed foods. Drink as much water as you can all day long to flush away bloating. Drink ice-chilled water and you'll burn a few extra calories as your body works to warm it up. Also, keep your diet balanced, eating a healthy ratio of carbohydrates, fats, and proteins. And, keep in mind, calories do count.
- Finally, train your abdominal muscles by simply keeping them contracted when performing all your other exercises, and when sitting, standing, or driving. Consciously holding them in can reduce back strain and help to flatten your entire midsection.

8.   How do I count calories?

Eat small portions. If you read the package, you know to stay away from trans fats, and if you continue to read the package, it will tell you how many calories are in the food. The average intake is 1,500 calories a day.

Also, watch your servings, basically back to small portions versus consuming the entire plate; don't count calories, I don't have time, too much work. Once again, I watch what I eat. Also, watch your condiments too; this is really tricky. Choose wheat bread rather than white bread; low-fat dressing, butter, mayonnaise etc., rather than regular condiments.

9. Do my genes have anything to do with my weight?

Yes, they do but that should not be an excuse. It just means you may have to work extra hard to reach your goals. The key is to gain weight naturally while exercising and toning your body at the same time. This way you ward off the extra pounds.

10. What is the best exercise for my thighs?

The best exercise is lying down on your side and doing the scissors exercise.

11. Does a Diet Coke really work with my double cheese-burger?

No, no, no, and NO!

12. How much should I eat?

You should eat as much as you want; you just have to be aware of your calorie in take, the types of food you eat, and most of all, drink plenty of water and exercise at least thirty minutes for three days a week.

13. How do I train my stomach to take in a little bit of food when I am used to gorging myself?

I eat really slowly and I watch the servings. After a while, you will know exactly how much to put on your plate. Once you get in the habit, you will begin to eat small portions and not go back for seconds. It is also important to eat a well-balanced meal, which could include chicken, fish, green vegetables, and a starch.

14. What is the best diet food?

There is no best diet food; just stop being greedy!

15. When should I push away from the table?

After you have had one plate of food—and only one plate of food. This is especially true at all-you-can-eat buffets, not to mention during holiday parties and gatherings with your family.

16. When should I skip dessert?

Never skip dessert; just share with someone else. Actually, once you have disciplined yourself, down to your desired weight, and exercising daily, dessert will not blow you up. Just remember, everything in moderation.

Losing Weight and Exercising – Myths and Facts

Fact: It takes the body seven minutes to realize your stomach is full; not realizing this, I ate slowly for years and did not realize what I was doing. I take about forty-five minutes to eat!

There are a lot of myths about losing weight; I am not surprised everyone gets confused. This book does not have all the answers, but it will definitely help you to differentiate between myth and fact.

Myth: If you drink a lot of water (more than recommended), you will get fat.

Facts: Natural water has absolutely no calories, so it can't be converted to fat. Actually, water dissolves fat. Besides, water is vital for the proper functioning of your body. If there is a relation between drinking much water and weight, it is a very indirect one, and water can't be blamed for that. When you drink water and it stays in your body, it's absolutely logical that your weight will be higher; but after a couple of hours, when water normally leaves your body, you will not have more fat.

Myth: Exercise makes you eat more.

Facts: Sure, when you exercise, you lose energy, but that does not mean that right after going out of the gym you must head to the restaurant. Experts often recommend that you neither eat nor drink gallons of water for at least two hours after physical activity. So if you don't eat after you have been exercising, you will not gain weight.

Myth: Diet alone is enough to lose fat.

Facts: Unfortunately, it is not as simple as that. After you have been on a diet for some time, even if there have been positive results, there is always a point when your body refuses to use more of its fat reserves and you can't lose a gram more. At this point, or, even better, from the very beginning, you must include exercise, because diets alone can't burn enough fat.

Myth: There are magic diets and pills.

Facts: Too good to be true. Magic diets that tell you that if you eat one thing, or don't eat this and this, you will have the body of a goddess, are really naïve. And, aside from keeping your mind busy through the day, other positive results are unlikely. The same applies to pills. Unless you have a serious metabolic disorder, which is a medical condition and needs to be treated by doctors, pills are the lazy way to great body.

LOSING WEIGHT AND EXERCISING - MYTHS AND FACTS

Myth: When you exercise hard, you can eat whatever you like.

Facts: This is the opposite of the dieting myth, but the grain of truth is the same. Even when you exercise hard (two or more hours a day), you still need to take into account what you eat and when you eat it. Two hours of active exercising might burn enough fat, but if you have a giant pizza and a huge bottle of Coke after that, forget about the positive effects of the gym—you will still have fat (though presumably more muscles as well).

Myth: You can lose fat only in a particular region of your body.

Facts: People with thin legs and a fat belly, or the opposite, are like this not because they want it, but rather because this is their body structure (which they probably don't like at all). When you lose fat, this happens in a pre-defined order. First, fat disappears from the face and the breasts. The belly and the hips come next. The thighs and the upper-arm usually are the last ones affected and, for many women, these areas never become fat-free.

Myth: Diets and exercise are universal.

Facts: People are different and diets and exercise are exceptions. While there are universally true facts about dieting and exercise, more often than not, successful and sustainable fat loss is achieved when you work hard at combining diet and exercise tailored to your needs.

Myth: You can lose fat once and forever.

HOW TO STAY SLIM ONE BITE AT A TIME

Facts: This hardly ever happens, though there are cases when one has been fat during puberty and as an adult his or her weight is in the norm. But for adults, losing fat means a constant struggle to maintain the achievements, so you can't rely on the idea that you will make some effort, drop your excessive weight, and then there will be no need to do anything.

Acknowledgements

I have been asked how do I stay so slim, well the answer is One Bite at a time!

During my early years my mom would serve dinner and dessert every night. I was very active in sports during this time.

As I got older I could no longer eat this way. Even though I literally at one bite at a time and still active, I had to watch the portions and what I was eating one bite at a time.

I realized the buck stopped here, I had to change my mindset, my eating habits, the time I ate, and the way I used to eat had to be revised. I would say to myself you mean to tell me I can not eat like I used to. I have always been slim, but now I had to learn "How to stay Slim"!

So in this book, I have written Common sense tips and the 16 most questions I get asked. I hope these tips can be an inspiration to a lot of people.

I would like everyone to know it is not as hard as you think.

Staying healthy and eating right will result in a better looking you and a healthier body.

Remember control your mind, you can control your eating habits

Author Biography

I would consider myself a fair person; I like equality, I believe in giving people the benefit of the doubt when other doesn't think twice about it. I grew up in a loving environment with my dad and mom, sister and brother. We did not have much but we had loving parents, who taught us right from wrong. Yes, I hit a few speed bumps but I got over them and believed these life lessons made me the person I am today. I love reading and writing. I often think of being surrounded by books, reading about new and exciting things every day. I always dreamed of reading a book a day! I just wanted to share a few tips with everyone who struggles with weight loss, eating right, and exercising. I would like everyone to know it is not hard as you think. I hope these tips can be an inspiration to a lot of people. It's not about the weight or shape; it is about staying healthy. Staying healthy and eating right will result in a better looking you as well as your body.